the healthy brain kit
workbook

SOUNDS TRUE

SOUNDS TRUE is a registered trademark of
Sounds True, Inc.
Boulder CO 80306

© 2007 Body & Soul Omnimedia, Inc. publisher of *Dr. Andrew Weil's Self Healing* newsletter
For subscription information, please call (800) 523-3296.

Portions of this workbook have been excerpted from
The Memory Bible by Gary Small, M.D., © 2002 Gary Small, M.D.
The Memory Prescription by Gary Small, M.D., © 2004 Gary Small, M.D.
The Longevity Bible by Gary Small, M.D., © 2006 Gary Small, M.D.
Reprinted by permission of Hyperion. All rights reserved.

Printed in China

ISBN 978-1-59179-530-8

contents

introduction

Who doesn't want a healthier brain? We all want a brain that thinks clearly, works quickly, and concentrates intently throughout the years. We also want an agile mind capable of storing and processing vast amounts of information, from the everyday (your shopping list, the punch line to a joke, your ATM PIN number) to the complex (balancing your checkbook, learning to tango, speaking Japanese). But while some people's brains seem to have a natural capacity for remembering sports statistics, television trivia, or historical facts, most of us recognize that there's some room for improvement where our cognitive capabilities are concerned.

No matter what your current situation is, the tips and techniques in *The Healthy Brain Kit* will be a good first step toward improved mental fitness and better brain health. Maybe you're interested in this kit because your memory isn't quite what it used to be, or because you're hoping to keep your mind in good working order as you age. Either way, you don't have to be an Ivy League grad, a member of Mensa, or a whiz at doing the *New York Times* Sunday crossword puzzle to benefit from the lifestyle advice and memory techniques you'll be learning.

In *The Healthy Brain Kit*, two well-known preventive-medicine physicians and best-selling authors—Andrew Weil, M.D., and Gary Small, M.D.—have teamed up to bring you a complete program of tools and teachings for boosting your brain health immediately. Whether you're concerned about forgetfulness, poor concentration, a lack of creativity, or you just want to regain the cognitive edge of your youth, *The Healthy Brain Kit* will give you the skills to keep your brain in optimum shape today and in the years ahead.

First, Dr. Weil will teach you how to lead a brain-protective lifestyle—from suggestions for diet and physical activity to relaxation techniques and a discussion of supplements that will help your mind stay sharp. Staying mentally fit requires effort. Dr. Weil writes in his latest book, *Healthy Aging* (2005, p. 226), "I am not at all convinced that cognitive decline is an inevitable consequence of aging. Rather, I think most people simply do not give themselves the kinds of mental challenges that brains need to retain their functionality."

Next, Dr. Small will lead you through a series of fun mental workouts to jump-start your brain, stretch your imagination, and strengthen your memory.

These exercises are designed to protect your brain so you retain your mental faculties for as long as possible. In his book *The Memory Prescription* (2004, p. 7), Dr. Small acknowledges that what matters most as we get older is not merely the quantity of years but the quality of life. He writes, "Medical science is striving to keep us alive for 120 years, but what's the point if you can't enjoy that longevity with a mentally fit brain?"

A HEALTHY-BRAIN ACTION PLAN

By following the six steps in this section, you'll safeguard your brain against the changes aging can bring and make the best use of this interactive learning kit.

1. Understand how your brain works. After reading this introduction to the workbook, read Section One: Your Amazing Brain. You'll become better acquainted with your brain, the way it works, and how aging might affect its abilities—positively, negatively, or not at all.

2. Assess your memory. Complete the subjective- and objective-memory tests in Section One to rate your current abilities. There's no need for test anxiety; these assessments are a guide—not the last word on your memory skills.

3. Adopt a brain-healthy lifestyle. Improving brain health involves more than solving puzzles and mastering memory techniques; it's also about discovering a sensible way to live your life. Everything from making good dietary choices and staying in shape to getting enough sleep and managing stress can have positive payoffs when it comes to your mental well-being.

4. Exercise your mind. Warm up your brain for the challenging workout ahead by doing several of the relaxation methods taught on CD One, Track 8, and CD Two, Tracks 3 and 4. You'll receive step-by-step instruction in stress-reducing techniques that will help you clear out mental clutter, calm down, and unwind tense muscles—techniques that will leave you feeling refreshed and

ready to optimize the capacity or your memory. Then begin your brain training by learning the three basic memory skills: *look, snap,* and *connect.* You'll have plenty of opportunities to practice these techniques through the exercises on CD Two, in the workbook, and on the brain-training cards. When you're ready, move on to the mental-aerobics exercises for a fun change of pace and to flex your brain in new and different ways. Finally, tackle the advanced memory techniques to build your skills and confidence.

5. Retest your memory skills. After you've spent time listening to the CDs, reading the workbook, and using the practical tools for at least two weeks, check your progress. Retake the subjective-memory assessment in this workbook and see if your score has improved. With your newfound mental prowess, you'll be well on your way to a healthier brain.

6. Keep at it. Take every opportunity to learn something new and stay mentally active. Seek out intellectually stimulating activities—from taking vacations in interesting locations and managing do-it-yourself home-improvement projects to researching your genealogy and pursuing creative outlets. If you're a fan of word puzzles, step out of your comfort zone and attempt math brain teasers instead. As you gain skills over time, expand your mental horizons by pursuing a higher degree of difficulty or more advanced techniques. With persistence, practice, and patience, you will have everything you need to keep your brain young, fit, and cognitively strong throughout life.

your amazing brain

Your brain is one amazing organ. It weighs a mere three pounds and is about the size of your two fists pressed together. It lets you think, speak, plan, remember, imagine, dream, and feel emotions. It gives you the power to reason, make decisions, and solve problems. It makes sense of the information coming in from your five senses. It controls your movements and posture, and regulates blood pressure, heart rate, and breathing without your conscious effort. To a great extent, your brain determines who you are.

With its one hundred billion neurons (nerve cells) and the one thousand *trillion* connections among them, the human brain is the most complex object in the known universe. The wrinkles and folds on the brain increase its surface area within the skull. The organ has a pinkish hue from the tiny blood vessels supplying it with oxygen and nutrients. The brain is composed primarily of water (78 percent), fat (10 percent), and protein (8 percent), and one brain surgeon has compared its consistency to soft tofu.

Each half, or hemisphere, of the brain—right and left—controls the opposite side of the body. In general, the left hemisphere is considered more logical, analytical, and objective, while the right hemisphere is thought to be more intuitive, creative, and subjective. (For more on the left and right brains, see page 37.) Different areas within each hemisphere are responsible for particular brain

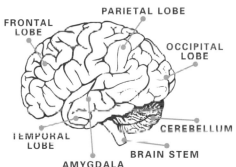

FRONTAL LOBE

PARIETAL LOBE

OCCIPITAL LOBE

CEREBELLUM

TEMPORAL LOBE

AMYGDALA

BRAIN STEM

functions. The frontal lobe plays important roles in planning, movement, and speech. The temporal lobe is involved in hearing and memory. The parietal lobe deals with pain and touch sensation, as well as spatial orientation. The occipital lobe handles vision, while the cerebellum is involved in balance, coordination, and movement. Finally, the brain stem transmits messages to and from the spinal cord, and regulates automatic body functions like breathing, blood pressure, and heart rhythm.

HIS BRAIN, HER BRAIN

There are several differences between the male and female brain that influence its anatomy and function but make little difference when it comes to general intelligence.

	MEN	WOMEN
size of brain	Bigger	Smaller
average weight	3 pounds	$2^2/_3$ pounds
key differences	Higher percentage of white matter (where the networking or connections between the information centers of the brain are located; composed of nerve fibers)	Higher percentage of gray matter (where the information-processing centers in the brain are located; composed of cell bodies)
advantages	May explain why men tend to have better visual and spatial abilities	May explain why women tend to have better language and verbal skills; brain possibly more efficient, meaning it takes less mental activity or work to perform the same task

6

BRAIN CHANGES DURING AGING

A slight slowing of thought and memory normally occurs with aging. This is due not so much to a loss of brain cells (the number of neurons lost over time is relatively small), but rather to changes that slow down the communication between brain cells. For instance, the levels of certain neurotransmitters (chemical messengers) decrease with age, and some neurons may have fewer dendrites (branches) to receive messages from neighboring cells. However, such changes shouldn't have a *major* impact on your life. (Severe memory loss and dementia are not normal and may be signs of Alzheimer's or other neurological diseases.)

Scientists long believed that once you reached adulthood, you stopped growing new brain cells. But now we know that new brain cells *do* form throughout life, even though you don't

replace all the cells you lose. One particularly encouraging finding is that the hippocampus—the most important brain structure for memory—regularly generates new brain cells.

HOW AGING DOES—AND DOESN'T—AFFECT MEMORY

Age-related changes in the brain tend to affect your memory and other cognitive functions in different ways. Here's a look at which functions are more vulnerable to aging and which are more resilient, according to *The Harvard Medical School Guide to Achieving Optimal Memory* (Nelson 2005, pp. 50–52).

More Affected by Age

- Ability to hold information temporarily in mind (working memory), such as hearing a phone number and then dialing it or comparing the price per ounce of two items

- Speed of processing information, which can affect retrieval of the names of acquaintances as well as your ability to keep pace in conversations
- Attention to detail, so that when you learn new information, you may take in the big picture or gist as well as a younger person, but you might not remember as many details
- Remembering verbal facts, such as names of people, places, and objects
- Remembering spatial information, such as the directions to a new location
- Recalling the location, date, and time of a specific event
- Multitasking

Less Affected by Age

- Ability to focus and sustain attention
- Knowledge of words, their meanings, and how to combine them in meaningful ways
- Skills and procedures for doing things, such as riding a bicycle or playing the piano
- Reasoning
- Willpower
- Creativity

MEMORY CHANGES: WHAT'S NORMAL AND WHAT'S NOT

The symptoms of Alzheimer's disease are more than simple memory lapses. Here are some differences between normal age-related memory changes and possible warning signs of Alzheimer's worth bringing to your doctor's attention.

NORMAL	NOT NORMAL
You occasionally forget names or appointments.	You forget recently learned information.
You occasionally forget why you came into a room or what you planned to say.	You have trouble performing familiar tasks. You lose track of the steps to prepare a recipe, place a phone call, or play a game.
You sometimes have trouble finding the right word.	You forget simple words or use unusual phrases like "that thing for my mouth" instead of "toothbrush."
You sometimes forget the day of the week or where you were going.	You get lost in your own neighborhood, or forget where you are or how you got there.
You temporarily misplace your keys or wallet.	You put an iron in the freezer or a wristwatch in the sugar bowl.

Source: Alzheimer's Association

BETTER WITH AGE?

Do some aspects of brain function improve with age? According to psychiatrist and gerontologist Gene Cohen, M.D., Ph.D., director of The Center on Aging, Health & Humanities at George Washington University, the answer is yes. In his book *The Mature Mind: The Positive Power of the Aging Brain* (2005, pp. 5–8, 14–23), he describes a number of beneficial changes.

- **Wiser.** Older brains have learned more than younger brains, and learning creates new connections between neurons. Although the neurons may lose some processing speed with age, they become more richly intertwined, reflecting both deeper knowledge and better judgment.

- **More flexible.** Unlike younger adults, who tend to handle most tasks on one side of the brain or the other, older people are more apt to use both sides at once. This adaptation not only helps keep you sharp, but may also help explain why autobiographical writing and storytelling are common among older people. The rearrangement of brain functions "makes it easier to merge the speech, language, and sequential thinking typical of the left hemisphere with the creative, synthesizing right hemisphere," suggests Dr. Cohen (2005, p. 23).

- **Greater equanimity.** The amygdalas, two almond-shaped structures that serve as the brain's emotional centers, appear to mellow with age. In brain-imaging studies, older adults show less evidence of fear, anger, and hatred than young adults. Likewise, psychological studies show that older adults are less impulsive and less likely to dwell on negative feelings.

CONDITIONS AND DRUGS THAT CAN INFLUENCE MEMORY

Alzheimer's disease and normal aging aren't the only causes of memory changes. Certain conditions (such as alcoholism, anxiety, depression, diabetes, hypertension, hypothyroidism, sleep disorders, and vitamin B-12 deficiency) can impair your ability to think and remember. If you're having memory problems, your doctor may advise a medical workup to determine if one of these conditions is responsible.

Meanwhile, be aware that medications can also affect memory. Such medications include anti-anxiety drugs, antidepressants, antihistamines, antispasmodics, beta-blockers for hypertension, cimetidine (Tagamet) for ulcers, narcotic painkillers, Parkinson's disease drugs, sleeping pills, and various forms of chemotherapy. If you suspect a medication is interfering with your memory, talk to your doctor about adjusting your dose or switching to another drug.

rating your memory abilities

You likely have a certain awareness of your memory abilities from moment to moment. Sometimes you might notice that you're doing better or worse on learning new information or recalling it. Other times friends and family members might comment on your forgetfulness or memory strengths. While these subjective observations can heighten your awareness of your memory abilities, there are standardized questionnaires that can help measure them.

Dr. Small and his UCLA research group have studied how these standard measures of memory self-awareness compare with objective measures (for example, how well a person can actually remember information on a written test), and self-assessments do reflect such true memory measures. These scientists also have found that self-assessments of memory correlate with how effectively neurons communicate when measured by brain scans.

Although many factors can influence these self-ratings—including mood, energy levels, and personality—memory questionnaires can provide a reasonable measure of memory ability. Based on his clinical practice and research at UCLA, Dr. Small has developed the following subjective-memory assessment for this program, which can provide a measurable guide to your true memory changes as well as other subtle aspects of brain function.

Using a pencil, answer the following questions by circling the number between one and seven that best reflects how you judge your own memory abilities. When you tally the results of your completed questionnaire, you will have a baseline of your current memory self-ratings—your "before" scores. Then take the test again at least two weeks after you have been practicing the memory techniques and lifestyle approaches taught in this program. Those self-ratings will be your "after" scores. Compare your results to gauge your improvement.

SUBJECTIVE-MEMORY QUESTIONNAIRE

	BAD		GOOD		GREAT	
How good is your memory now compared with when you were young?	1	2	3	4	5	6	7
How good is your memory compared with that of other people your age?	1	2	3	4	5	6	7
In general, how would you rate your memory ability throughout life?	1	2	3	4	5	6	7

How much do each of the following memory tasks or events challenge you?

	OFTEN		SOMETIMES		RARELY	
Keeping appointments	1	2	3	4	5	6	7
Remembering names and faces	1	2	3	4	5	6	7
Knowing where you put your glasses or keys	1	2	3	4	5	6	7
Recalling what someone told you	1	2	3	4	5	6	7
Keeping track of birthdays	1	2	3	4	5	6	7
Recalling words you rarely use	1	2	3	4	5	6	7
Recalling words you often use	1	2	3	4	5	6	7
Walking into a room and forgetting why	1	2	3	4	5	6	7
Losing track of what you're saying	1	2	3	4	5	6	7
Misplacing papers or objects you're carrying	1	2	3	4	5	6	7
Other people commenting that you're repeating yourself	1	2	3	4	5	6	7
Losing track of where you're driving	1	2	3	4	5	6	7
Forgetting where you parked your car	1	2	3	4	5	6	7

How good is your memory for
events that occurred ...

	BAD	AVERAGE	GREAT
Several hours before	1 2	3 4 5	6 7
The day before	1 2	3 4 5	6 7
Several weeks ago	1 2	3 4 5	6 7
Several months ago	1 2	3 4 5	6 7
Several years ago	1 2	3 4 5	6 7

	OFTEN	SOMETIMES	RARELY
How often do other people comment about your everyday memory challenges?	1 2	3 4 5	6 7
How often do you worry about your memory challenges?	1 2	3 4 5	6 7

Add up all the numbers you have circled and write in your sum below.

Subjective-Memory Total Score, Baseline _____

INTERPRETING YOUR SCORE

TEST SCORE	RESULT
130 or higher	Your subjective-memory difficulties are minimal.
70 to 129	You might be noticing a slight to moderate degree of memory change.
Below 70	You might be experiencing an even greater self-awareness of memory difficulties.

Whatever your score on this first assessment, this simply represents your baseline—once you've worked with the contents of this program, your score should go up.

ASSESSING YOUR OBJECTIVE MEMORY

On CD Two, Dr. Small offers you several opportunities to check your objective-memory abilities by recalling lists of words. Each of these tests is a briefer version of a more extensive assessment that his research group uses in their work at the UCLA Memory and Aging Research Center.

In parts one and three of the memory assessment, you will be asked to remember a list of eight words, which will be read to you slowly. Then, in parts two and four of the memory assessment, you will be asked to revisit, in your own memory, the list of words you have just learned—and to see how many you can recall. After you have taken each assessment, write down the total number of words you can recall in the appropriate blanks that follow.

MEMORY ASSESSMENT, PART TWO
Objective-Memory Total Score, Baseline _____

MEMORY ASSESSMENT, PART FOUR
Objective-Memory Total Score, Baseline _____

TEST SCORE	RESULT
Six or above	You will likely find the basic memory skills easy to master and can quickly move on to more advanced techniques.
Less than six	Spend more time learning basic memory skills before moving on.
Less than three	No need to panic; this program can help improve your scores. If not, consider speaking with your physician about your memory abilities.

Factors such as your age and level of education can influence your objective-memory score (younger people and those with more education typically score better). Remember, your results are an indicator or guide—not the last word—regarding your current brain fitness.

TIP A common cause of memory complaints is worry and anxiety about performance—and for good reason. Worry about memory difficulties may indeed worsen your objective-memory performance.

SECTION THREE
adopting a brain-healthy lifestyle

from Andrew Weil, M.D.

n ot so long ago, scientists regarded memory problems and cognitive decline as inevitable consequences of aging. I'm pleased this view is changing, as more and more studies show that you can take steps to preserve your memory and keep your mind sharp throughout life. What's more, it now appears that genetics account for only one-third of an individual's risk of developing Alzheimer's disease. Your environment and the lifestyle choices you make on a day-to-day basis account for two-thirds of the risk, giving you more control over your brain's future health than you may have thought possible.

The earlier in life that you adopt brain-protective practices, the better, since the abnormal protein deposits (amyloid plaques) and tangles of nerve fibers that accumulate in the brains of Alzheimer's patients may begin forming decades before symptoms first appear. Dietary and other lifestyle measures can address several factors that undermine brain health, including chronic inflammation (Alzheimer's begins with inflammation in the brain), oxidative stress from free radicals, and chronically elevated levels of the stress hormone cortisol. Healthy living can also help prevent cardiovascular disease, an all-too-common problem that can reduce blood supply to critical areas of the brain and frequently contributes to dementia.

Even your attitude toward aging can affect your memory: older people who were shown negative words about aging, like *senile,* before taking memory tests did worse than those who were shown positive words, like *wisdom.* Likewise, in China and other cultures with a more positive view of aging than ours, older people performed better on memory tests.

The following lifestyle strategies can help you protect your brain's health. Remember, the more of these you practice and the sooner you incorporate them, the healthier your brain will be.

MENTALLY EXERCISING YOUR BRAIN

Engaging your brain appears to be a key protective strategy. The more education you have, the less likely you are to experience age-related cognitive decline or to develop Alzheimer's disease. If you do experience these conditions, they'll more likely appear later in life for you than for people with fewer years of education. The reason may have to do with "neural redundancy," the number of extra connections between nerve cells in the brain. Learning creates new connections between brain cells, and many of these connections duplicate existing pathways. The more connections you have, the more you can afford to lose if some degenerative process should occur.

An advanced degree isn't necessary. The important thing is to keep challenging your mind. A study of more than 450 adults aged seventy-five or older found that reading books and newspapers, playing cards and board games, doing crossword puzzles, playing a musical instrument, and dancing may all reduce the risk of Alzheimer's disease (Verghese et al. 2003).

Two of the best mental workouts I know of are learning to use a new computer-operating system and learning a new language. If you use a computer, you know the frustration associated with switching to a new operating system. But this is exactly the kind of mental challenge that forces the brain's neural network to change, to make more connections, and to stay flexible and young. Likewise, learning another language keeps you in a continual state of mental workout, in ways that are both frustrating and rewarding. One intriguing study suggests that being bilingual can help protect against age-related cognitive decline (Bialystok et al. 2004). This type of learning draws on "fluid intelligence," the ability to stay focused and to manage attention while ignoring irrelevant information. Fluid intelligence is one of the first aspects of brain function to suffer with advancing age, so having proficiency in two languages can be protective.

Learning memory-improvement techniques is another great way to sharpen recall. Later in this workbook and on CD Two, Dr. Gary Small will teach you some of the methods to improve memory and boost brain fitness that have proved effective in his research.

Could some activities dull the mind? A recent study of some three hundred older women found that those who watched daytime soap operas or talk shows were more likely to have cognitive impairments than women who skipped such programs. However, researchers say it's unclear whether watching these TV shows leads to weaker brainpower or vice versa (Fogel and Carson 2006).

27 marvelous mental workouts

Learning a new computer-operating system and learning a foreign language are two of the best ways to challenge your mind. Here are many more possibilities:

- Solve crossword, Sudoku, or jigsaw puzzles.
- Play cards, chess, word games (like Scrabble), and knowledge games (like Trivial Pursuit).
- Join a book club or study group.

- Express yourself by writing, painting, making music, or dancing.
- Attend lectures, plays, and concerts.
- Visit museums.
- Travel to new destinations.
- Volunteer for a cause you care about.
- Take classes at a local adult-education center or community college.
- Start a new hobby, whether it's collecting stamps, woodworking, or bird-watching.
- Do more math by making simple calculations in your head, balancing your checkbook without a calculator, or preparing your own taxes.

THE BRAIN-BOOSTING BENEFITS OF PHYSICAL ACTIVITY

A number of large studies show that older people who get regular exercise are more likely to keep their minds sharp. For example, a study of nearly six thousand women aged sixty-five or older found that those who walked the most blocks per week had a 34 percent lower risk of cognitive decline than those who walked the fewest blocks (Yaffe et al. 2001). Other research has found that exercise programs involving both aerobic exercise (like walking) and strength training produced better results on cognitive abilities than either activity alone. Exercise improves blood flow and oxygen delivery to the brain, and may spur the formation of new brain cells. For optimum health, I recommend that your exercise program include the following components:

Aerobic exercise is any activity that raises your heart rate and makes you breathe harder. Walking is the most popular aerobic activity, and for good reason. It requires no equipment, everyone knows how to do it, and it carries the lowest risk of injury. I suggest you walk briskly to make it aerobic. Other options include running, swimming, biking, playing tennis, skiing, dancing, and working out on elliptical trainers, treadmills, and stationary bicycles. Aim for thirty to forty-five minutes of aerobic activity at least five days a week.

Strength training works muscles against resistance in order to build and maintain bone and muscle mass. You can strength-train using weight machines, free weights, resistance bands, stability balls, and your own body weight by doing push-ups and squats. If you're new to this sort of activity, I advise working with a fitness expert who can teach you some basic techniques and show you how to do them safely. You'll want to strength train two or three days a week, taking at least one day off between sessions.

Flexibility and balance exercises can help you stay limber and loose. Whenever your body has been in one position for a while, it's good to stretch it in the opposite direction briefly. For instance, if you work at a desktop computer, get up periodically and do a gentle backward bend. Also, consider taking up yoga, tai chi, or qigong, three ancient Eastern disciplines that promote flexibility, balance, and relaxation. You can learn these disciplines in group classes or from private instructors, and then practice them at home using a video or DVD.

protecting your head from harm

A history of head trauma is linked to a higher risk of Alzheimer's disease, perhaps due to low-grade inflammation persisting after the injury has healed. To avoid sports-related head injuries, wear head protection when bicycling, skating, and skiing. Wearing a helmet while biking can reduce the risk of brain injury by nearly 90 percent, according to one study (Thompson et al. 1989). Other ways to protect your head include using a seat belt in your car, uncluttering your house to avoid falls, wearing protective headgear while riding on a motorcycle, and wearing shoes with good traction in slick weather.

FEEDING YOUR BRAIN AN ANTI-INFLAMMATORY DIET

Because inflammation and oxidative stress can undermine brain function, eating an anti-inflammatory diet that is rich in antioxidants and omega-3 fatty acids can help you keep your wits about you. To add "brain food" to your diet, you'll want to *consume more* of the following:

Fish. People who eat fish regularly are less likely to experience cognitive decline or develop Alzheimer's. The omega-3s in oily fish, such as salmon, sardines, herring, and black cod, help to reduce inflammation, and one of these healthy fats—DHA—is essential for normal brain function. Vegetarian sources of omega-3 fatty acids include walnuts, flax seeds (preferably freshly ground), and hemp seeds.

Fruits and vegetables. According to a 2004 analysis of more than one hundred foods by scientists at the U.S. Department of Agriculture (Wu et al. 2004), berries and beans have particularly high concentrations of antioxidants. (For a list of the top twenty foods, see page 24.) The pigments that account for the varied colors of vegetables and fruits have antioxidant properties, so it's a good idea to eat fresh produce every day from as many parts of the color spectrum as you can.

Olive oil. This monounsaturated fat contains an anti-inflammatory substance called squalene and antioxidant compounds such as flavonoids and polyphenols. Make extra-virgin olive oil your primary cooking oil: it's less processed than other kinds of olive oil and has more antioxidant activity.

Turmeric. The low rate of Alzheimer's disease in India may be partly due to daily consumption of turmeric there. The yellow spice, which is a major ingredient in Indian curries and American mustard, is a powerful anti-inflammatory agent. Consider flavoring more of your food with it.

Green tea. A recent study of some one thousand Japanese people aged seventy or older found that those who drank at least two cups of green tea a day were 54 percent less likely to have cognitive difficulties than those who had three cups or fewer a week (Kuriyama et al. 2006). The antioxidants in this beverage

did you know?
Between 50 and 60 percent of the brain's dry weight comes from fat.

are probably responsible for its brain-protective effects.

Meanwhile, you'll want to *limit* or *eliminate* foods that promote inflammation, which include the following:

Trans fats. Strictly avoid margarine, vegetable shortening, and all products listing them as ingredients, as well as all products made with partially hydrogenated oils.

Polyunsaturated vegetable oils. Avoid regular safflower and sunflower oils, corn oil, cottonseed oil, and mixed-vegetable oils.

Saturated fat. Reduce your intake by eating less butter, cream, cheese, and other full-fat dairy products, unskinned chicken, fatty meats, and products made with coconut and palm-kernel oils.

Wheat flour and sugar. Cut down on bread and packaged snack foods like chips and pretzels. Foods made with wheat flour and sugar tend to cause spikes in blood sugar, which foster abnormal reactions between proteins and sugars, resulting in pro-inflammatory compounds.

did you know? The brain's sole energy source is sugar (or glucose). Unlike other cells in the body, brain cells cannot convert fats or proteins into glucose.

top antioxidant foods

Here's a list of the top twenty food sources of antioxidants, based on their total antioxidant capacity per serving size (Wu et al. 2004).

1. Small red beans
2. Wild blueberries
3. Red kidney beans
4. Pinto beans
5. Blueberries (cultivated)
6. Cranberries
7. Artichoke hearts
8. Blackberries
9. Prunes
10. Raspberries
11. Strawberries
12. Red Delicious apples
13. Granny Smith apples
14. Pecans
15. Sweet cherries
16. Black plums
17. Russet potatoes
18. Black beans
19. Plums
20. Gala apples

PROTECTING YOUR BRAIN FROM STRESS

The stress hormone cortisol is toxic to nerve cells in the hippocampus (the part of the brain concerned with memory), so I strongly recommend incorporating a relaxation technique into your daily routine to keep stress—and cortisol—in check. You have many options. Yoga, tai chi, and qigong can release both physical and mental stress. Other relaxation techniques include:

Breath work. The Relaxing Breath exercise that I describe on CD One, Track 8 and on the brain-training card entitled The Relaxing Breath is one of the most cost- and time-efficient relaxation methods I know. In addition to practicing this exercise, it's a good idea to make your breathing slower, deeper, quieter, and more regular whenever you think of it. Slow, deep breathing delivers more oxygen to your brain and the rest of your body. Surprisingly, the best way to deepen respiration is by *exhaling* more air, not by inhaling more of it. Try taking a deep breath, letting it out effortlessly, and then squeezing out more air. You should feel the effort in the intercostal muscles between your ribs. If you squeeze out more air whenever you think of it, you'll gradually build up these muscles, and the length of your exhalations will naturally equal that of your inhalations. (In most people, inhalations last much longer.)

Meditation. In its most basic sense, meditation is simply focused attention, directed to the breath, a repeated word or phrase (known as a *mantra*), or a mental image. By keeping your attention in one place, you're also taking your focus away from anxious thoughts and the mental chatter that can often fill your head. You can practice meditation using the techniques on the brain-training card entitled Meditation Vacation. Meditation quiets the mind, and it may even slow brain deterioration related to aging.

In a recent study, brain regions involved in memory and attention were thicker in people who meditated regularly. While these areas tend to shrink with age, older meditators were able to ward off some of this shrinkage (Lazar et al. 2005).

Visualization. Both guided imagery and self-hypnosis take advantage of the power of visual imagination to promote relaxation. A basic technique of these approaches is to imagine an actual place from past experience where you've felt supremely happy, secure, and peaceful. Then you picture yourself in that scene, making all your sense impressions as sharp as possible. You'll practice this relaxation technique in the five-minute break on the brain-training card called The Break and on CD Two, Track 3. You can learn more about these approaches from books and audio programs or by working with a hypnotherapist or guided-imagery practitioner.

Progressive muscle relaxation. This mind-body technique, described on the brain-training card entitled Muscle Unwinder and taught by Dr. Small on CD Two, Track 4, involves gently and consciously tightening one muscle group at a time, followed by releasing this tension. You progressively move from head to toe or from the feet upward. The idea is to pay attention to how your body feels as you alternately squeeze and relax each major muscle group. When you're done, you'll feel relaxed all over.

KNOWING THE IMPORTANCE OF SOCIAL CONNECTIONS

Middle-aged and older adults with large social networks experience less cognitive decline as they age. People with an active social life may be more likely to stay involved in mentally challenging activities, and good social ties can be a powerful buffer against stress. Some experts believe that dancing may be particularly beneficial to the brain, because it combines social interaction, physical activity, and often the mental challenge of learning dance steps.

There are many other ways to stay connected. Spend time with family and friends, especially those who make you feel happier and more alive. Meet other people interested in healthy living by joining a walking or biking club or taking yoga or cooking classes. Consider getting involved at a local house of worship: there's some evidence that religious attendance and personal spiritual practices are associated with slower rates of cognitive decline. Do some kind of service work by volunteering in your community or helping someone in need. And think about getting a pet: caring for a companion animal can promote a sense of well-being, help manage stress, and make you smile.

OTHER LIFESTYLE FACTORS INFLUENCING BRAIN HEALTH

Here's how some other lifestyle choices can affect your brain's health:

Smoking. Heavy smokers are at much greater risk of developing cognitive impairment earlier in life than nonsmokers, perhaps as early as age fifty. Smoking interferes with blood flow and oxygen delivery to the brain, and it's a major risk factor for heart attack and stroke. (Nicotine itself may have some brain-protective properties, and pharmaceutical researchers are looking for analogs that lack the drug's harmful effects.)

Alcohol. Heavy alcohol consumption contributes to memory loss and increases the risk of Alzheimer's, but moderate alcohol consumption may help prevent dementia, perhaps by improving cardiovascular health. If you're under age sixty-five, moderate drinking means no more than one drink a day for women and no more than two drinks a day for men. Those aged sixty-five or older shouldn't have more than one daily drink.

Rest and sleep. Brain cells need downtime to process and store memory. In one study, volunteers who slept only four to six hours a night for fourteen consecutive days did as poorly on memory tests as those who were totally deprived of sleep for two consecutive nights. Surprisingly, they were largely unaware of how sleep deprivation was impairing their thinking and memory (Van Dongen et al. 2003). Although people vary in their need for sleep, many adults require seven to eight hours of sleep on most nights to perform at their mental peak.

Environmental toxins. Chronic, low-level exposure to environmental toxins like pesticides, herbicides, and heavy metals may increase the risk of Parkinson's disease and amyotrophic lateral sclerosis (ALS, or Lou Gehrig's disease). In a recent study, people who reported regular exposure to pesticides had a 70 percent higher incidence of Parkinson's than those who weren't exposed to the chemicals (Ascherio et al. 2006).

THE BEST SUPPLEMENTS FOR BRAIN HEALTH

In addition to getting antioxidants from your diet, I recommend beginning a daily antioxidant regimen to help protect your brain cells from the toxic effects of oxidative stress. I suggest you take the following every day:

- 200 mg of vitamin C
- 400 IU of natural vitamin E as mixed tocopherols (or 80 mg of mixed tocopherols and tocotrienols)
- 200 mcg of selenium
- 10,000 to 15,000 IU of mixed carotenoids

I also advise supplementing your diet with B vitamins (take a B-50 B-complex supplement or a multivitamin) to lower blood levels of homocysteine. High levels of this amino acid—which is formed in the breakdown of dietary protein, especially animal protein—are associated with lower cognitive function. And if you aren't eating oily fish at least twice a week, take a fish-oil supplement providing one to two grams of EPA and DHA combined per day.

Some people report benefits from "smart" supplements. I'll discuss three of the more promising ones here. All are available at health-food stores and on the Internet, and ginkgo is now sold over the counter in most drugstores.

Ginkgo. This extract from the leaves of the ginkgo tree (*Ginkgo biloba*) increases blood flow to the head and has been shown to slow the progression of dementia in early-onset Alzheimer's disease. Although ginkgo is widely used as a memory booster,

I believe it is useful only for people with impaired circulation to the brain (due to atherosclerosis, for example). Look for extracts standardized to contain 24 percent ginkgo flavone glycosides and 6 percent terpene lactones, and take 60 to 120 mg twice a day with food. It may take six to eight weeks of use to produce an effect.

Acetyl-L-carnitine. Also called ALC, this amino-acid derivative is involved in the production of energy in the mitochondria, the power plants of all cells, including brain cells. ALC also helps the body make the memory-promoting neurotransmitter acetylcholine. Some preliminary evidence suggests that the combination of ALC and alpha-lipoic acid (ALA), such as in Juvenon, may slow the progression of Alzheimer's disease, particularly among younger patients, and may slow age-related cognitive decline not associated with Alzheimer's. The dose for ALC is 500 to 1,000 mg twice a day on an empty stomach. ALC with or without ALA is nontoxic but can be expensive. (The combination of ALA and ALC in Juvenon also helps stabilize blood sugar. I like this combination and take it myself.)

Phosphatidylserine. This naturally occurring fat is a component of the membranes that cover brain cells. Phosphatidylserine (PS) supplements, derived from soybeans, may be helpful for treating age-associated memory impairment, and they also hold promise for slowing the progression of early Alzheimer's disease. (There is less evidence that PS enhances mental function in healthy people under fifty.) PS can be pricey, with some products costing $1 or more per day. A typical starting dose is 100 mg, two or three times a day. If this produces benefits after a month or more, you can try going on a lower maintenance dose of 100 or 200 mg daily. PS may have a blood-thinning effect, so talk with your doctor before trying it if you take anticoagulant medications.

maximizing your memory skills

from Gary Small, M.D.

the condition of your memory may be a telling sign of the health of your brain. Some memory loss is normal. From time to time, you might draw a blank on the name of a familiar face, misplace your keys or eyeglasses, or forget why you walked into a room. When you're in your twenties, thirties, or forties, you might laugh off these memory lapses, or chalk them up to stress or distraction. People aged fifty or over often joke about their memory mishaps and label them as "middle-age pauses" or "senior moments." Using humor can mask an underlying fear of the mental decline seen in some older adults. If memory mishaps seem to occur more frequently, it may be a good idea to seek medical advice to rule out any physical brain problems. But forgetting is not necessarily a symptom of a disease, a sign of senility, or an inevitable aspect of getting older—memory is a skill that can simply get rusty over time. The good news is that the memory techniques you'll be learning in *The Healthy Brain Kit* can help keep your brain in great shape and enhance your memory abilities.

The methods you'll be learning on CD Two, in this workbook, and on the thirty-five brain-training cards are the same tools I use with my own patients at the UCLA Memory Clinic. Between the memory-training techniques I'm about to share and the lifestyle advice Dr. Weil has given you, you have at your fingertips all the resources you need to maintain a young and vital mind and to maximize your mental performance.

As I wrote in my latest book, *The Longevity Bible* (2006, p. 23), "Memory defines who we are, now and at every moment. It also defines our future, because without memory ability, we cannot make plans and think ahead. And, of course, without memory, it's as if we have no past. Staying mentally sharp requires optimum memory performance, the foundation of any quality longevity program."

Evidence suggests that memory-training programs work. In the first study of its kind, carried out at the UCLA Memory and Aging Research Center, people improved their cognitive function and brain efficiency by making the kinds of lifestyle changes described in this program, such as including physical activity, sensible eating, stress reduction,

did you know?
There is no such thing as a truly photographic memory—there are only people with exceptionally good memory techniques.

and memory exercises in their daily lives. Researchers looked at seventeen people aged thirty-five to sixty-nine with mild self-reported memory complaints. Half were assigned to a two-week healthy-lifestyle program that involved practicing twenty minutes of daily mental exercises, as well as getting regular physical activity and eating a healthy diet, while the others made no lifestyle changes. After fourteen days, those in the healthy-lifestyle group had significant changes in brain efficiency in the area that controls everyday memory tasks, or "working memory," while the control group showed no significant changes (Small et al. 2006).

HOW MEMORY WORKS

How does information get filed away into your memory? Learning is the first step to remembering anything. When you're awake, your senses are bombarded with stimuli, such as sights, sounds, and other sensations that are all potential memories. These pass through your *immediate memory* into a holding area known as *short-term memory*. Most of these are fleeting sensations lost in a few milliseconds, but of the few retained in short-term memory, only a small percentage ever make their way into *long-term memory* storage. The kind of information that gets stored in short-term memory may include the name of someone you just met or what you ate for breakfast. When you have trouble remembering something, it's often because you weren't concentrating, were distracted, or didn't learn it very well in the first place—and not necessarily because you can't recall the information.

BASIC MEMORY TRAINING

Look, snap, and *connect* are the three foundational steps of the memory techniques you will learn in this program.

Look reminds you to focus your attention, especially when new information is presented.

Consciously absorb the details and meanings from a new face, event, or conversation. The most common explanation for memory loss is that the information never gets into your mind in the first place, usually because you are distracted, not interested, or multitasking. *Look* is a skill that involves all five senses, not just vision; hearing, smell, touch, and taste also contribute to effective learning.

Snap reminds you to create a mental snapshot or visual image of the information to be remembered. As you picture this image in your mind's eye, add details to give the snapshot personal meaning—and thus make it easier to learn and recall later.

Connect calls for linking up the visual images in a relational and meaningful way.

These relationships are the key to drumming up memories when you want to recall them later. The ideas or images become part of a chain, starting with the first item, which is associated with the second, and so on.

Now let's put these basic skills into practice.

look: actively observe what you want to learn

Take out several frequently used objects (such as keys, eyeglasses, and a hairbrush), place them on a table, and stare at them, one at a time. Pay attention to details you never noticed before. You will find quite a few.

TIP Think of your brain as a sponge—you want to absorb as many details as possible to augment your memory skills.

snap: create mental snapshots of memories

Visualize each of the following but alter them slightly so they become unusual in some way.

• Football   • Rock star   • Orange   • Car

TIP To help develop effective learning and recall techniques, you need to rekindle the natural creative instincts you had as a child.

connect: linking up mental snapshots / exercise 1

For each of the following four objects, create a vivid, detailed, and personally meaningful image. Connect these images by creating a story that links them sequentially.

• Athlete   • Animal   • Drink   • Antique

TIP If you need to remember a long list of items, the link method is an elaborate way to connect mental snapshots by creating a story. The story's visual images and flow provide the cues for retrieving information.

---

connect: linking up
mental snapshots / exercise 2

For each of the following word pairs, imagine a situation or an activity that involves the two words together and that is reasonable or logical in some way.

- Lion / Tree
- Paddle / Net
- Cart / Horse
- Cruise ship / Swimming pool

Now go back to the word pairs above and imagine a bizarre or illogical linkage for each

TIP The more vibrantly and creatively you visualize new information, the more effectively it will stick in your memory. Exaggeration and playfulness enhance your ability to store and recall information.

AEROBICIZING YOUR MIND

Mental aerobics are tasks or exercises that involve a mental challenge. They can take many forms, from completing a crossword or Sudoku puzzle to reading an engrossing novel. The aim of these exercises is to shake up your usual mental assumptions and force you to think of novel solutions. And by doing so, these workouts help stretch, tone, and strengthen your brain. Choose activities that you enjoy and that seem fun, whether it's learning a musical instrument or solving jigsaw puzzles. No one form of mental exercise has been shown to be more effective than another, so let your personal preferences be your guide. Remember, mental-aerobics exercises should only be challenging enough to stimulate the brain without stressing it.

Just as physical activity can keep your body strong, mental activity can keep your mind sharp and agile. Experts believe that one reason why solving puzzles and other forms of mental stimulation help to lower the risk of dementia is that people develop a "cognitive reserve" that allows them to tolerate more damage from Alzheimer's and other brain diseases. In one study of nearly 470 older adults, people who were the most mentally active had a 63 percent lower risk of getting dementia compared with those who rarely read, played board games, or did similar leisure activities (Verghese et al. 2003). In other studies, people who had been intellectually active in their forties and fifties were three times less likely to develop Alzheimer's than those who

did you know?
Brain teasers and puzzles often involve lateral thinking, which means you are trying to solve a problem from many angles instead of tackling it head on.

hadn't been. In fact, more mental activity among twenty-somethings led to a more promising outlook for cognitive function later in life. One Columbia University scientist, Yaakov Stern, Ph.D. (2003), has concluded that it's not how much brain you have, but how you use it, that makes the difference.

CROSS-TRAINING YOUR BRAIN WITH MENTAL AEROBICS

Ideally, in a mental-stimulation program, you want to work both hemispheres (or sides) of your brain to strengthen it. For right-handed people, the right side of the brain controls spatial relationships and the left side specializes in verbal skills and logical analysis. For lefties, the hemisphere functions listed here are reversed.

LEFT-BRAIN FUNCTIONS	RIGHT-BRAIN FUNCTIONS
Logical analysis (reasoning, drawing conclusions)	Spatial relationships (reading maps, doing jigsaw puzzles)
Information sequencing (making lists, organizing thoughts)	Artistic and musical abilities
Language and speech	Face recognition
Reading and writing	Depth perception
Counting and mathematics	Dreaming
Symbol recognition	Emotional perception
	Sense of humor

In this program, puzzles and teasers are sometimes labeled according to the hemisphere that tends to work the hardest when you're trying to answer them. One goal of mental aerobics is to work both sides of the brain, so it's good to alternate right-brain exercises, such as mazes and map reading, with left-brain activities, such as verbal and logic skills.

TIP Whenever you push yourself to solve problems in a new way, you may be strengthening the connections between brain cells.

MENTAL AEROBICS: INTERMEDIATE

left-brain exercise

Starting with the word "warm" and using only letters from the final word "file," change one letter at a time until you have the word "file." Each word must result in a proper word.

Warm _____ _____ _____ File

Answer: Warm, Farm, Firm, Film (or Fire), File

left-brain exercise

See how many words you can spell from the letters below. No letter may be used twice, and each word must have the letter "h" in it.

H　　S　　E　　R　　C　　A　　O

Answer: Arch(es), ash, cash, chase, chore(s), chose, crash, hare(s), has, he, hear(s), ho, hoe(s), hose, rah, rash, reach, roach(es), search, share, she, shear, shoe, shore.

whole-brain exercise

Count the number of F's in the following sentence: "Fresh fish is an excellent source of omega-3s and a better source of antioxidants than many realize."

Answer: There are four; many people don't process the word "of."

MENTAL AEROBICS: ADVANCED

left-brain exercise

Which is the odd one out?

- Grouper
- Catfish
- Tuna
- Angelfish

Answer: Catfish is the only freshwater fish. All the others are saltwater fish.

whole-brain exercise

Fill in the boxes so that you spell out the following words either horizontally or vertically.

Amen   Ends   Lend   Mate   Mole   Omen   Tend

Answer:

whole-brain exercise

Fill in the grid so that every row, column, and three-by-two box contains the digits 1 through 6. It's best to use a pencil with an eraser.

1		2	6		
	5			1	
2	6	4			
				4	6
			1		
5	2			6	3

Answer:

1	3	2	5	6	4
4	5	6	3	1	2
2	6	4	5	3	1
3	1	5	2	4	6
6	4	3	1	2	5
5	2	1	4	7	3

GETTING ORGANIZED IMPROVES BRAIN EFFICIENCY

Your brain has only a limited amount of memory capacity, so it's important to be selective about what information you want to remember. Using external memory tools can help give you greater brain efficiency. These external memory tools can help you become more organized, and poor organizational skills may be the reason why you have difficulty remembering to begin with. Some indispensable organizational techniques include the following:

Effective notes. Writing something down helps to reinforce information in your memory. Note taking is not only good for classroom-style learning. You might also want to jot down a new business idea you have, a question to ask your doctor, a book you'd like to read, or a restaurant you want to try. You can also write down important things you need to know occasionally, such as how to program the VCR or change your computer password.

Memory places. Put commonly misplaced items in the same "memory" place, such as your car keys on a hook near the door, your daily organizer in the same pocket of your briefcase, and your scissors in a particular desk drawer.

Daily planning lists. Whether for work, grocery shopping, or other errands, making lists helps you keep track of tasks that need to be done. When you complete a task, cross it off. Lists can be prioritized by deadline, or you can place an asterisk by items that require immediate action or attention.

Weekly or monthly planning calendars. These help you to record and keep track of regular or occasional appointments, events, or meetings.

Date books, electronic organizers. These portable devices help track the details of your life; electronic versions can hold a variety of organizational tools, such as calendars, address books, and to-do lists, providing easily accessible information.

Post-it notes. These stick-on notes are perfect for written reminders, making them a good quick-fix as an external memory aid and visible cue.

Memory habits. You learned some in childhood, like brushing your teeth every morning and before bed. These habits, such as always placing your car keys in a certain spot or using an alarm clock, can augment your other memory aids.

Daily routines. Adding structure to your life in the form of regular routines in your daily schedule helps to free up time for focusing on other things you wish to do or learn.

MASTERING ADVANCED MEMORY TECHNIQUES

In order to become a memory master, you must also master the skill of organization. Organization is the process of systematically arranging information according to patterns, structures, and groups. Learning to organize information effectively facilitates quick memory storage and retrieval. Many accomplished individuals credit some measure of their memory success to their organizational skills.

TWO MENTAL-ORGANIZATION EXERCISES

grouping words together: exercise 1

Group the following twelve items into three categories:

Pool	Punch line	Facsimile
Memo	Pond	Jibe
Pun	Lagoon	IOU
Lake	Post-it	Gag

Answer: To group the items, you need to recognize the categories: paperwork (facsimile, memo, Post-it, IOU), bodies of water (pond, lagoon, pool, lake), and jokes (pun, jibe, punch line, gag).

grouping words together: exercise 2

Group the following twelve items into three categories:

Yarn	Drawer	Vial
Tobacco tin	Suture	Lentil
Pepper	Shoebox	Wick
Cocoa	Licorice	Dental floss

Answer: To group the items, you need to recognize the categories: edibles (pepper, cocoa, licorice, lentil), stringy objects (yarn, dental floss, suture, wick), and containers (tobacco tin, drawer, shoebox, vial).

One of the most effective organizational memory skills involves *chunking*—dividing information into smaller groups or clusters. It's easier to remember three chunks of three- or four-digit numbers than an entire ten-digit phone number.

using chunking to recall numbers

Memorize your driver's license ID by chunking the numbers together.

Look up a phone number from your personal phone book and chunk the numbers into groups of two, three, and four.

remembering names and faces

The main reason why you may forget names, sometimes seconds after being introduced, is that you're not fully listening. But you can use *look, snap, connect* to remember them. Make sure you consciously listen to the name (*look*), then *snap* a visual image of the name and face, and finally *connect* the name and face.

1. For practice, look at the names below and think of a visual image.

NAME   VISUAL IMAGE

Stewart   _____

Cheryl   _____

2. Now that you're warmed up, write down the last name of two people you know and create a mental snapshot that represents their name.

NAME   VISUAL IMAGE

_____   _____

_____   _____

3. For the above people, list the first distinguishing feature that comes to mind.

NAME   FEATURE NAME / FACE IMAGE

_____   _____

_____   _____

The process of thinking up the images and making the connections, or links, will help fix these names into memory.

THE PEG METHOD FOR REMEMBERING NUMERICAL SEQUENCES

Just as a peg is something that pins down or fastens things, this technique helps you to systematically pin down or fasten bits of information. It's a system developed for remembering numerical sequences, such as phone numbers and addresses, by visualizing objects instead of rotely memorizing the numbers themselves. Pegging increases the possibility that the information will make it into your long-term memory stores, but it requires effort.

To use the Peg Method, you will need to commit to memory ten specific, simple visual images—one for each of the ten numerical digits. For example, you may use the image of a tie to represent the number one because the outline of a tie looks like the number one.

Here is an example of some sample peg images you might use for each of the ten digits. You can learn and use these images or make up your own pegs.

NUMBER	IMAGE	MEMORY AID
1	Tie	A necktie looks like the number one
2	Tooth	"Tooth" sounds like "two"
3	Thread	"Three" sounds like "thread"
4	Fork	"Fork" sounds like "four"
5	Snake	A curved snake looks like the number five
6	Sax	"Sax" sounds like "six"
7	Walking stick	A walking stick with a handle looks like the number 7
8	Eight ball	The "8" on an eight ball reminds you of the number 8
9	Knife	"Knife" sounds like "nine"
0	Zebra	The first letter of "zero" and "zebra" is "z"

practicing the peg method

To remember the phone number 555-0217, use the pegs to create a story with the following sequence of pegs: snake-snake-snake-zebra-tooth-tie-walking stick.

Example: The story you might create with these pegs could go something like this: Three snakes slide up to a zebra whose tooth has just fallen out onto his necktie. He uses his walking stick to push it back into place.

MAKING THE MOST OF MEMORY TRAINING

By now, you've realized that memory training can be an empowering way to boost your brain health and your confidence. If you challenge yourself and commit to using these tools in your everyday life, you will see a difference. As you begin using these techniques on a more regular basis, keep these seven do's and don't's of memory training in mind.

Do start simple. Begin with simple mental-stimulation exercises and move up to more complex ones. Keep building your level of challenge over time, and continue to learn new things.

Don't strain. Find mental challenges that are fun and engaging, but not ones that are so tough that you *strain*, rather than *train*, the brain. You want a level of mental challenge that keeps you interested without frustrating or exhausting you.

Do assign personal meaning and detail to information you want to remember. Doing so will help get information to your memory faster and allow it to stay there longer.

Don't multitask too much. This can actually make you less, rather than more, productive. You might not remember things as well when you're trying to manage several details at the same time. Too much multitasking can lead to increased stress, anxiety, attention deficits, and memory loss.

Do get enough sleep. You need sufficient shut-eye to give your brain the downtime it needs for effective memory consolidation. Without adequate sleep, you might lack energy and alertness, and may feel "fuzzy-headed" or confused the next day. Insomnia and fatigue are major sources of stress that can impair concentration and memory.

Don't stress out. Find some relaxation techniques that work for you to release stress. Stress and the hormones that go with it interfere with your ability to learn and recall information as well as to concentrate, and many researchers believe that prolonged periods of stress may accelerate brain aging and age-related memory decline.

Do have fun. These techniques can really stimulate your imagination, so experiment with them and have fun!

resource guide

Here are some valuable resources to learn more about brain health, memory training, aging well, and other essential skills to keep your body and mind in good working order.

FROM DR. SMALL AND DR. WEIL
Books

The Memory Bible: An Innovative Strategy for Keeping Your Brain Young by Gary Small, M.D. (Hyperion, 2002)

The Memory Prescription: Dr. Gary Small's 14-Day Plan to Keep Your Brain and Body Young by Gary Small, M.D., with Gigi Vorgan (Hyperion, 2004)

The Longevity Bible: 8 Essential Strategies for Keeping Your Mind Sharp and Your Body Young by Gary Small, M.D., with Gigi Vorgan (Hyperion, 2006)

Healthy Aging: A Lifelong Guide to Your Physical and Spiritual Well-Being by Andrew Weil, M.D. (Knopf, 2005)

Recordings

Improve Your Memory Now with Gary Small, M.D. (Sounds True, 2003)

Improve Your Memory with Gary Small, M.D. (Sounds True, 2005). This program is excerpted from *Improve Your Memory Now.*

Breathing: The Master Key to Self Healing with Andrew Weil, M.D. (Sounds True, 1999)

Dr. Andrew Weil's Guide to Optimum Health (Sounds True, 2002)

Kits

Dr. Andrew Weil's Mind-Body Tool Kit (Sounds True, 2005). A great resource to lower the stress that can impair your memory and harm your brain, this kit includes 2 CDs, a 52-page workbook, and 25 mind-training cards to help you practice breath work, meditation, guided imagery, and sound therapy.

To learn about the university center that Dr. Small directs, contact:
UCLA Center on Aging
10945 Le Conte Avenue, Suite 3119
Los Angeles CA 90095-6980
(310) 794-0676
www.aging.ucla.edu

OTHER RESOURCES
Books

Age-Proof Your Mind: Detect, Delay, and Prevent Memory Loss—Before It's Too Late by Zaldy S. Tan, M.D., M.P.H. (Warner Wellness, 2006)

The Better Brain Book: The Best Tools for Improving Memory and Sharpness and Preventing Aging of the Brain by David Perlmutter, M.D., and Carol Colman (Riverhead Trade, 2005)

The Female Brain by Louann Brizendine, M.D. (Morgan Road Books, 2006)

The Harvard Medical School Guide to Achieving Optimal Memory by Aaron P. Nelson, Ph.D., with Susan Gilbert (McGraw-Hill, 2005)

Intelligent Memory: Improve Your Memory No Matter What Your Age by Barry Gordon, M.D., Ph.D., and Lisa Berger (Penguin Books, 2004)

Keep Your Brain Young: The Complete Guide to Physical and Emotional Health and Longevity by Guy McKhann, M.D., and Marilyn Albert, Ph.D. (John Wiley & Sons, 2003)

The Mature Mind: The Positive Power of the Aging Brain by Gene D. Cohen, M.D., Ph.D. (Basic Books, 2005)

The Seven Sins of Memory: How the Mind Forgets and Remembers by Daniel L. Schacter (Houghton Mifflin, 2002)

The Wisdom Paradox: How Your Mind Can Grow Stronger as Your Brain Grows Older by Elkhonon Goldberg, Ph.D. (Gotham Books, 2005)

WEB SITES

To learn more about living a brain-healthy lifestyle, visit:
www.aarp.org/health/brain
http://alz.org/maintainyourbrain/overview.asp
www.drweil.com

To do mental aerobics and brainteasers, visit:
www.brainbashers.com
www.greylabyrinth.com
www.dse.nl/puzzle/index_us.html
www.aarp.org/fun/puzzles

To stay informed about the latest research on the mind and the brain, visit:
www.drgarysmall.com
www.sciencedaily.com/news/mind-brain

ORGANIZATIONS

To find a medical specialist who can care for patients
with neurological disorders, contact:
American Academy of Neurology
1080 Montreal Avenue
St. Paul MN 55116
(800) 879-1960 or (651) 695-2717
www.aan.com

To find a health professional dedicated to
enhancing the mental health and well-being of older
adults, contact:
American Association for Geriatric Psychiatry
7910 Woodmont Avenue, Suite 1050
Bethesda MD 20814
(301) 654-7850
www.aagpgpa.org

about the authors

Andrew Weil, M.D., received an A.B. degree in biology (botany) from Harvard University and his M.D. from Harvard Medical School. He is director of the Program in Integrative Medicine, professor of public health, and clinical professor of medicine at the University of Arizona in Tucson. Dr. Weil is an internationally recognized expert on medicinal herbs, mind-body interactions, nutrition, and integrative medicine. He was named one of *Time* magazine's 100 most influential people of 2005. His ten books include *Healthy Aging, Eating Well for Optimum Health, 8 Weeks to Optimum Health,* and *Spontaneous Healing.* He is also editor of a monthly newsletter, *Self Healing* (www.selfhealing.com), and editorial director of a popular Web site, www.drweil.com. In addition, he is director of integrative health and healing at Miraval Life in Balance Resort near Tucson

Gary Small, M.D., is the chief of the UCLA Memory and Aging Research Center and a professor of psychiatry and biobehavioral sciences at the Semel Institute for Neuroscience and Human Behavior. For his work in the prevention of Alzheimer's disease and brain aging, *Scientific American* magazine named him "one of the world's top 50 innovators in science and technology." Dr. Small is the author of *The Memory Bible, The Memory Prescription,* and *The Longevity Bible.* He lectures extensively all over the world and often appears on national television shows, including *20/20, Good Morning America,* the *Today* show, CNN, *NBC Nightly News,* and *CBS News.* His work has been featured in the *New York Times, Wall Street Journal, Los Angeles Times, Washington Post, Time, Newsweek,* and *USA Today.* He also has a Web site, www.drgarysmall.com.

works cited

Ascherio, A., et al. 2006. Pesticide exposure and risk for Parkinson's disease. *Annals of Neurology* 60 (2): 197–203.

Bialystok, E., et al. 2004. Bilingualism, aging, and cognitive control: Evidence from the Simon Task. *Psychology and Aging* 19 (2): 290–303.

Cohen, Gene D. 2005. *The Mature Mind: The Positive Power of the Aging Brain*. New York: Basic Books.

Fogel, J., and M.C. Carson. 2006. Soap operas and talk shows on television are associated with poorer cognition in older women. *Southern Medical Journal* 99 (3): 226–33.

Kuriyama, S., et al. 2006. Green tea consumption and cognitive function: A cross-sectional study from the Tsurugaya Project. *American Journal of Clinical Nutrition* 83 (2): 355–61.

Lazar, S.W., et al. 2005. Meditation experience is associated with increased cortical thickness. *NeuroReport* 16 (17): 1983–87.

Nelson, Aaron P., with Susan Gilbert. 2005. *The Harvard Medical School Guide to Achieving Optimal Memory*. New York: McGraw-Hill.

Small, G.W., et al. 2006. Effects of a 14-day healthy longevity lifestyle program on cognition and brain function. *American Journal of Geriatric Psychiatry* 14 (6): 538–45.

Small, Gary, with Gigi Vorgan. 2006. *The Longevity Bible: 8 Essential Strategies for Keeping Your Mind Sharp and Your Body Young*. New York: Hyperion.

Small, Gary, with Gigi Vorgan. 2004. *The Memory Prescription: Dr. Gary Small's 14-Day Plan to Keep Your Brain and Body Young*. New York: Hyperion.

Stern, Y., et al. 2003. Exploring the neural basis of cognitive reserve. *Journal of Clinical and Experimental Neuropsychology* 25 (5): 691–701.

Thompson, R.S., et al. 1989. A case-control study of the effectiveness of bicycle safety helmets. *New England Journal of Medicine* 320 (21): 1361–67.

Van Dongen, H.P., et al. 2003. The cumulative cost of additional wakefulness: Dose-response effects on neurobehavioral functions and sleep physiology from chronic sleep restriction and total sleep deprivation. *Sleep* 26 (2): 117–26.

Verghese, J., et al. 2003. Leisure activities and the risk of dementia in the elderly. *New England Journal of Medicine* 348 (25): 2508–16.

Weil, Andrew. 2005. *Healthy Aging: A Lifelong Guide to Your Physical and Spiritual Well-Being*. New York: Alfred A. Knopf.

Wu, X., et al. 2004. Lipophilic and hydrophilic antioxidant capacities of common foods in the United States. *Journal of Agricultural and Food Chemistry* 52 (12): 4026–37.

Yaffe, K., et al. 2001. A prospective study of physical activity and cognitive decline in elderly women: Women who walk. *Archives of Internal Medicine* 161 (14): 1703–08.